Lose The Fat Now

<u>DISCLAIMER</u>

TABLE OF CONTENT

INTRODUCTION:

The problem of excess body weight and obesity has become a growing concern in the modern world. According to recent studies, more than 2 billion adults worldwide are overweight or obese. This condition not only affects one's physical appearance but can also lead to severe health problems such as diabetes, heart disease, and stroke. Therefore, it is essential to maintain a healthy weight and reduce excess fat in the body. In this guide, we will discuss various ways to lose the fat now and lead a healthy life.

CHAPTER 1: UNDERSTANDING BODY FAT

Before we talk about how to lose fat, it is important to understand what body fat is and why it is harmful. Body fat is a natural substance found in the body that stores energy. It is essential for maintaining body temperature and cushioning organs. However, when the body stores too much fat, it can lead to health problems. Excess body fat can increase the risk of heart disease, high blood pressure, stroke, and diabetes.

Although the term "fat" is often used to refer to all body fat, your body contains a variety of different forms of fat.

Some fats may be harmful to your health and aid in the development of disease. Others are advantageous and required for your wellness.

White, brown, and beige cells are the three major colors of fat cells. They could be kept in visceral, subcutaneous, or vital fat.

Every kind of fat has a specific purpose. Some support normal hormone and metabolic levels, whereas others support the development of fatal disorders, such as:

cardiovascular disease, excessive blood pressure, and cancer
Keep reading to figure out more about the various kinds of body fat.

WHITE FAT

Most people first consider white fat when thinking of fat. It is made up of big, white cells that are kept in the thighs, arms, buttocks, and belly, either under the skin or close to the organs. By storing energy in these fat cells, the body can use it later.

Also, this kind of fat is very important for the way certain hormones, like:
Leptin and estrogen (one of the hormones that stimulates hunger)
hormonal insulin (a stress hormone)

Despite the fact that some white fat is important for health, too much of it is exceedingly hazardous. Depending on how fit or active you are, there are different healthy body fat percentages.

Men who are non-athletes should have a total body fat percentage in the 14 to 24 percent range, while women should be in the 21 to 31 percent range, according to the American Council on Exercise.

The following health problems can put you at danger if your body fat percentage is higher than recommended:

Diabetes type 2
Cardiovascular disease
Blood pressure is high.
Pregnancy problems
Hormone abnormalities, and stroke
Renal illness
Cancerous liver disease

BROWN FAT

Although adults do still maintain a very little amount of brown fat, particularly in the neck and shoulders, brown fat is mostly seen in infants.

To keep you warm, this type of fat burns fatty acids. To help prevent obesity, researchers are interested in learning how to increase brown fat's activity.

BEIGE (BRITE)

The study of beige (or brite) fat is a relatively recent development. Between brown and white fat cells, these cells perform intermediate functions. Similar to brown fat, beige cells can aid in fat burning as opposed to storing it.

It's thought that specific hormones and enzymes generated under stressful situations, cold weather, or physical activity can aid in the transformation of white fat into beige fat.

This is an important field of research since it may help minimize obesity and increase amounts of healthy body fat.

ESSENTIAL FAT

For your life and a healthy body, necessary fat is just that—important. You have this fat in your:
brain bone marrow nerves organ-protecting membranes
Vital fat is crucial in the regulation of hormones, particularly those that govern temperature regulation, vitamin absorption, and reproduction.

Women need at least 10 to 13 percent of their body composition to come from essential fat, while men need at least 2 to 5 percent, according to the American Council on Exercise.

SUBCUTANEOUS

The fat deposited beneath the skin is referred to as subcutaneous fat. It consists of white, beige, and brown fat cells.

Our bodily fat is primarily subcutaneous. It's the fat on your arms, abdomen, thighs, and buttocks that you can pinch or squeeze.

Fitness experts estimate the proportion of total body fat by measuring subcutaneous fat with calipers.

A certain amount of subcutaneous fat is normal and beneficial, but too much can affect hormone sensitivity and balance.

VISCERAL

Visceral fat, commonly referred to as "belly fat," is the white fat that is kept around all of your major organs, including the liver, kidneys, pancreas, intestines, and heart, and is stored in your abdomen.

Your risk for diabetes, heart disease, stroke, vascular disease, and several malignancies can all be exacerbated by high levels of visceral fat.

BENEFITS

The constitution of the body is crucial. A healthy total fat percentage will improve your body's performance. Many advantages come from maintaining a healthy body fat percentage, such as:

- Temperature control
- Improved reproductive health, regulated hormone levels, and appropriate vitamin storage
- Optimum brain function
- A sound metabolism
- Normal blood sugar

RISKS

Visceral fat, in particular, can be hazardous to your health if you have too much white fat. You are more likely to have the following health issues if you have visceral fat:

Heart condition

Stroke

Cardiovascular disease

Problems from pregnancy and atherosclerosis

Type 2 diabetes affects hormones and causes various malignancies.

CHAPTER 2: CAUSES OF EXCESS BODY FAT

The causes of excess body fat are multifactorial. Some of the most common causes include a sedentary lifestyle, poor diet, hormonal imbalances, genetics, and certain medications. In this chapter, we will discuss each of these factors in detail and how they contribute to the accumulation of body fat.

OBESITY:

Obesity is a chronic, multifactorial condition that can result in excessive body fat and, occasionally, poor health. Of course, excess body fat itself is not an illness. Yet, an excessive amount of additional body fat might alter how your body works. These changes are gradual, have the potential to get worse over time, and may have a negative impact on health.

The good news is that by reducing part of your excess body fat, you can reduce your health risks. Your health can be significantly impacted by even slight weight fluctuations. Every weight loss strategy does not work for everybody.

Most people have made multiple attempts to lose weight. And maintaining a healthy weight is just as crucial as losing it initially.

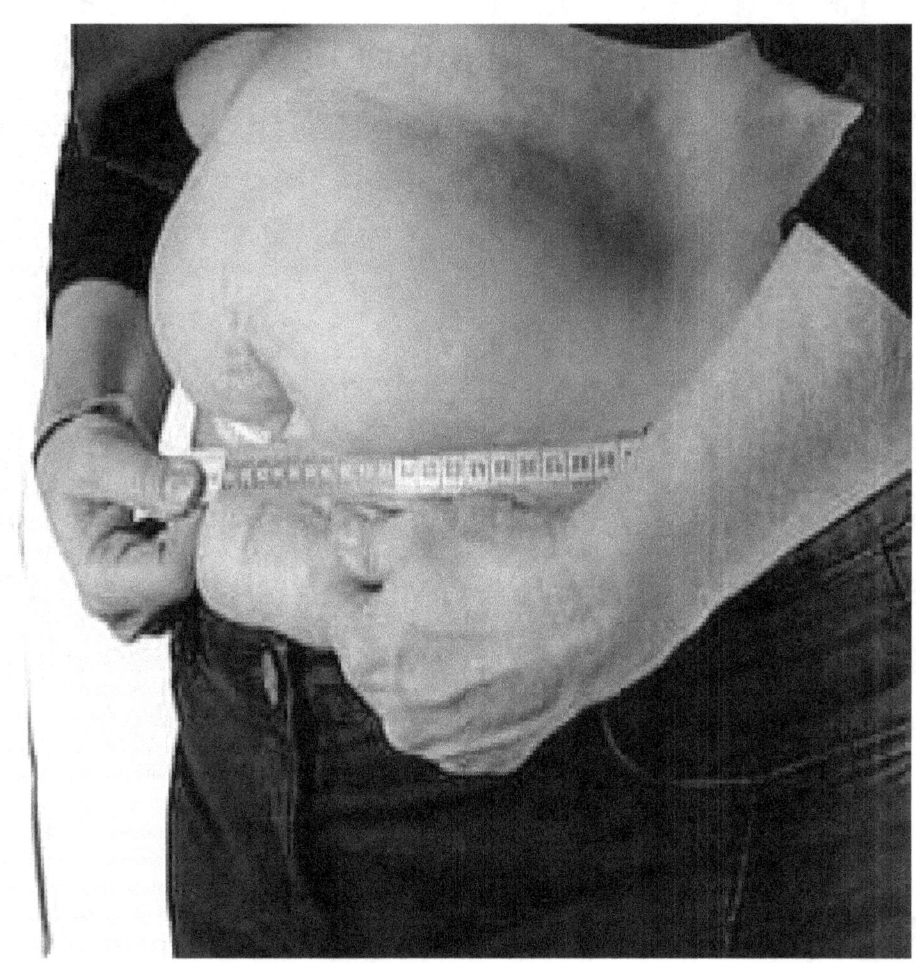

IS OBESITY A WEIGHT-BASED CONDITION?

The Body Mass Index (BMI) is frequently used by healthcare professionals to categorize obesity in the general population. The BMI calculates the ratio of average body weight to average height. Healthcare professionals often consider a BMI of 30 or higher to be obese. Although BMI has its limitations, it is a simple measure that can help you become aware of the health concerns associated with obesity.

Limitations include people like bodybuilders and athletes, who may have higher BMIs despite having low amounts of body fat because they have greater muscle. At a "normal" weight, obesity is also a possibility. You could be at the same risk for health problems as someone with a higher BMI if your body weight is average but your body fat percentage is high.

Healthcare professionals have also noted ethnic variations in the amount of excess weight that individuals may carry before it compromises their health. Black people are more likely to have health hazards at a higher BMI than Asian people, for instance, while Asian people are more likely to have health problems at a lower BMI than Black people.

The measurement of waist circumference is another method of evaluating obesity. According to statistics, you are more likely to develop problems linked to obesity if you have more body fat around your waist. When your waist measures greater than 35 inches for persons assigned female at birth or 40 inches for people assigned male at birth, the risk becomes high.

WHAT THREE FORMS OF OBESITY ARE THERE?

Depending on how severe illness is, healthcare experts categorize obesity into different class categories. They perform it using BMI. Your BMI is considered to be between 25.0 and 29.9 kg/m2, which is considered overweight. Healthcare professionals examine which therapies might be the most effective for each patient using three main categories of obesity. They consist of:

- **Obesity class I: BMI 30 to 35 kg/m2.**
- **BMI 35 to 40 kg/m2 is considered class II obesity.**
- **Obesity class III: 40 kg/m2 or higher BMI.**

WHAT IS MORBID OBESITY, EXACTLY?

Class III obesity is no longer referred to as "morbid obesity." "Morbidity" refers to linked health concerns in medical terminology. Class III obesity was referred to be "morbid" by doctors since it was most likely to be accompanied by concomitant health issues.
But, due to its negative implications, they decided to retire the phrase.

HOW IS KID OBESITY EVALUATED?

Medical professionals calculate children's obesity using BMI, but they do it in relation to the child's age and assigned sex. If a child's BMI is more than 95% of their peers in the same group, they may be labeled with obesity if they are older than 2 years. Depending on the population they are sampling, different growth charts may show slightly different BMI averages.

HOW BEING OBESE IMPACT YOUR BODY

Your body is impacted by obesity in various ways. Some of these consequences of having extra body fat are purely mechanical. For instance, it is easy to distinguish between more weight on your body and added strain on your joints and skeleton. More subdued impacts include blood chemistry changes that raise your risk for diabetes, heart disease, and stroke.

Certain consequences still need to be better understood. For instance, obesity increases the risk of developing some cancers.
 It exists, however we're not sure why. According to statistics, being obese raises your risk of dying young from any reason. Furthermore, studies demonstrate that reducing even a minor amount of weight (5% to 10%) can considerably lower these risks.

METABOLIC ADJUSTMENTS

Your metabolism is the process through which calories are transformed into energy to power various bodily processes. Your body turns excess calories into lipids and stores them in your adipose tissue when there are more calories than it can consume (body fat).

The size of the fat cells themselves increases when there is no longer any tissue in which to store lipids. Hormones and other substances that cause inflammation are secreted by enlarged fat cells.

The impacts of chronic inflammation on health are numerous. It influences your metabolism by causing insulin resistance, among other things. This indicates that your body can no longer effectively lower blood sugar and cholesterol levels with the help of insulin (sugars and fats in your blood). Elevated blood lipids and blood sugar (cholesterol and triglycerides)also contribute to high-blood pressure.

THE TERM "METABOLIC SYNDROME" refers to these risk factors taken together. They are combined because they all frequently reinforce one another. Moreover, they encourage continued weight gain and make it more difficult to lose weight and maintain weight loss. Metabolic syndrome is a common contributor to obesity and numerous disorders that are associated to it, such as:

- **DIABETES TYPE 2.** Obesity especially increases the risk of Type 2 diabetes by seven and twelve times, respectively, depending on the gender allocated at birth. For every additional point on the BMI scale, the risk rises by 20%. It also gets smaller as you lose weight.

- **CARDIOVASCULAR CONDITIONS.** Heart disease risk factors include high blood pressure, high cholesterol, high blood sugar, and inflammation. These conditions include coronary artery disease, congestive heart failure, heart attack, and stroke. Your BMI goes hand in hand with an increase in these hazards. Fatty liver disease is the greatest cause of preventable death both globally and in the United States. Your liver, which is in charge of filtering your blood, receives extra lipids that are circulating in your blood. The accumulation of extra fat in your liver can cause chronic liver inflammation (hepatitis) and long-term liver damage (cirrhosis).

- **KIDNEY DISEASES.** Among the most frequent causes of chronic kidney disease are high blood pressure, diabetes, and liver disease.

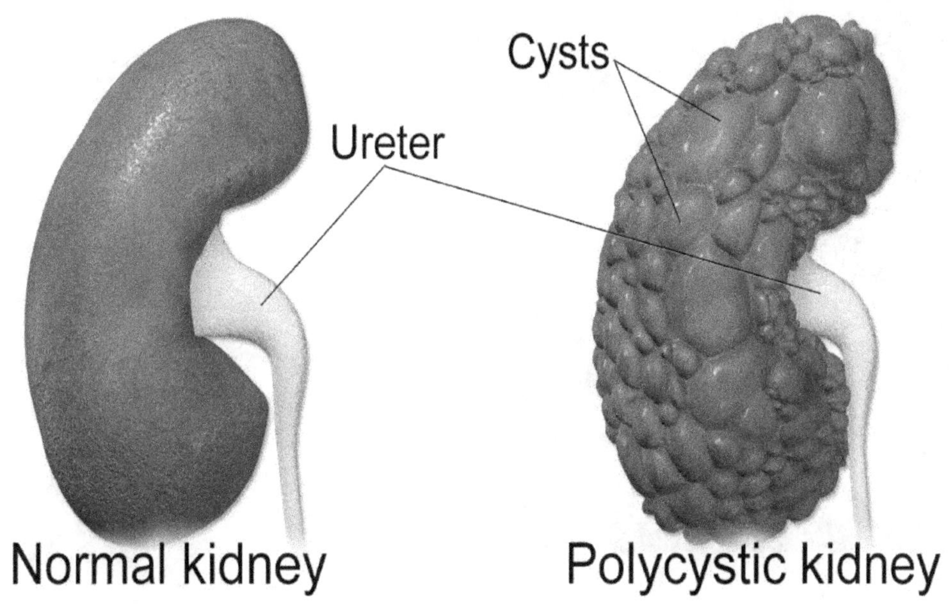

- **GALLSTONES.** Increased blood cholesterol levels can result in gallstones and other possible gallbladder problems by causing cholesterol to build up in your gallbladder.

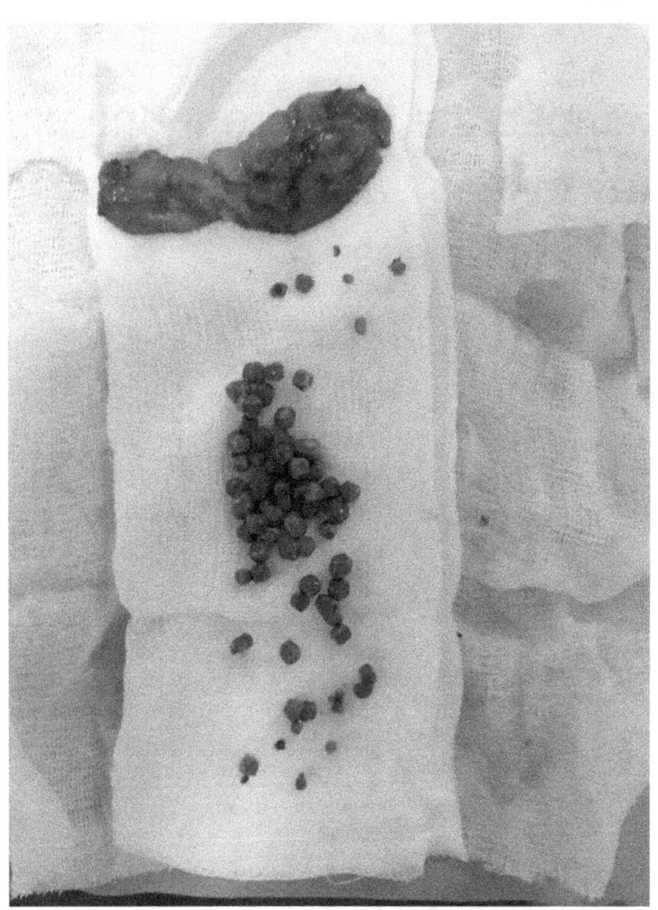

DIRECT EFFECT

The respiratory system's organs may become crowded by excess body fat, and your musculoskeletal system may experience tension and pressure. These things help:

- Asthma.
- Apneic sleep.
- the syndrome of obesity hypoventilation.
- Osteoarthritis.
- back ache.
- Gout.

The US Centers for Disease Control and Prevention report that 1 in 3 obese persons also have arthritis. According to studies, the likelihood of developing knee arthritis increases by 36% for every 5 kg you acquire. The good news is that a 10% weight loss combined with exercise can considerably lessen discomfort from arthritis and enhance your quality of life.

IMMEDIATE CONSEQUENCES

Moreover, obesity has indirect links to:

- Memory and cognition, including an increased risk of dementia and Alzheimer's disease.
- Problems during pregnancy and female infertility.
- depression and mental health issues.
- Esophageal, pancreatic, colorectal, breast, uterine, and ovarian malignancies are only a few examples.

WHY DOES OBESITY OCCUR?

Obesity is primarily brought on by consuming more calories than your body can utilize. Many elements play a role in this. Some elements are unique to you. Others are included into our society's framework on a global, regional, or family scale. In certain aspects, actively combating these various causes is necessary to prevent obesity.

The following variables may cause an increase in caloric intake:

FOODS THAT ARE QUICK AND EASY. It's simple to consume a lot of calories in communities and families where highly processed fast and convenience meals are dietary mainstays. These foods can make you feel more ravenous since they are lacking in fiber and other nutrients and heavy in sugar and fat. These components encourage compulsive eating behaviors.

They might represent in some communities due to price and accessibility, these can be the only food types that are easily accessible.

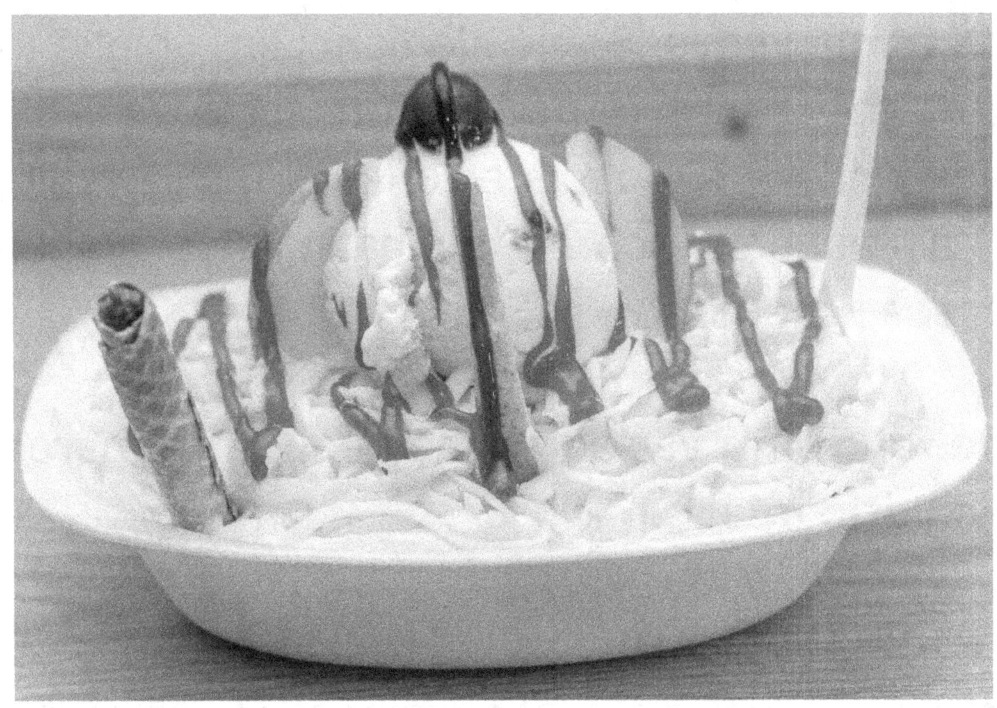

According to the Centers for Disease Control, 40% of American households are more than a mile away from a healthy food outlet.

EVERYTHING CONTAINS SUGAR. The food industry isn't set up to keep us healthy. It is intended to market goods that we will become dependent on and desire to purchase more of. Sweets and sugary drinks, which have little nutritional value and a lot of extra calories, are among the top things on that list. But even normal foods have large levels of added sugar to make them more tempting and addicting. It's so widespread that it has altered our standards for flavor.

ADVERTISING AND MARKETING. The items that we need the least but that the industry requires us to buy the most are processed foods, candies, and sugary drinks, which are heavily promoted by ubiquitous advertising. These products are presented in advertising as being commonplace and essential to daily life.

These products are presented in advertising as being commonplace and essential to daily life. Alcohol is sold largely through advertising, which contributes many empty calories.

PSYCHOLOGICAL DETERMINANTS. In today's environment, boredom, loneliness, worry, and sadness are all prevalent and can all cause overeating. These might encourage us to eat more of certain high-calorie food kinds that stimulate the pleasure centers in our brains. It's a basic human instinct to eat when we're feeling bad. Humans evolved to obtain food, and evolution hasn't kept up with the level of food abundance currently enjoyed by Western societies.

HORMONES. Our hunger and fullness cues are controlled by hormones. Many factors, including common ones like stress and sleep deprivation as well as uncommon ones like genetic variants, might impair these regulatory functions. Even when you don't need any more calories, hormones can make you keep wanting more food.
These may make it difficult to recognize your point of exhaustion.

CERTAIN MEDICINES. You may gain weight if you take medications to treat other diseases. Among these are beta-blockers, antidepressants, steroids, anti-epileptic drugs, and drugs for diabetes.
There are several elements that could reduce the amount of calories we burn:

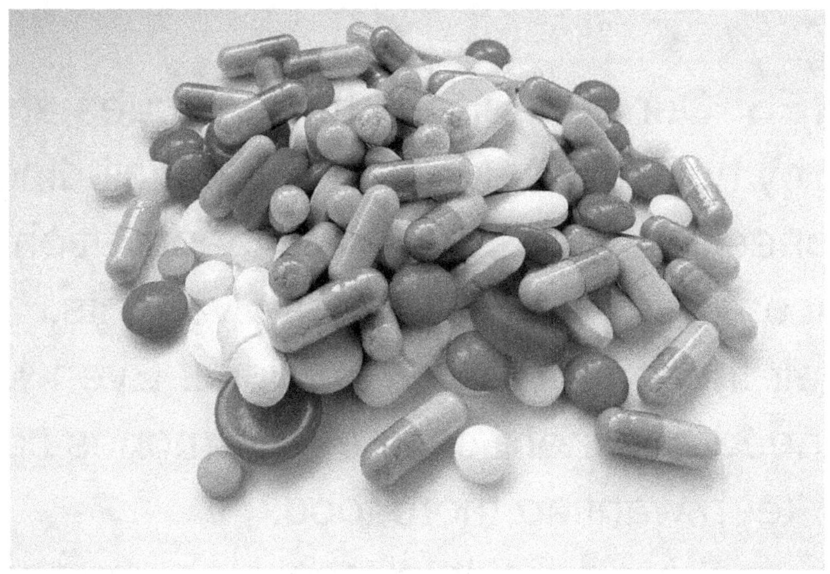

MEDIA CULTURE. We spend more time in front of our phones and computers as job, shopping, and social life move online. Long stretches of sedentary entertainment are more likely thanks to streaming media and binge-watching.
Workforce adjustments. More individuals today work at desks than on their feet as a result of industrial shifts that favor automation and computers. They put in longer hours as well.

WORKFORCE ADJUSTMENTS. More individuals today work at desks than on their feet as a result of industrial shifts that favor automation and computers. They put in longer hours as well.

FATIGUE. A snowball effect results from sedentary behavior. According to studies, sitting stationary for a prolonged period of time causes fatigue and demotivation. Sitting stiffens the body and causes aches and pains that limit movement. It also contributes to general tension, which increases tiredness.

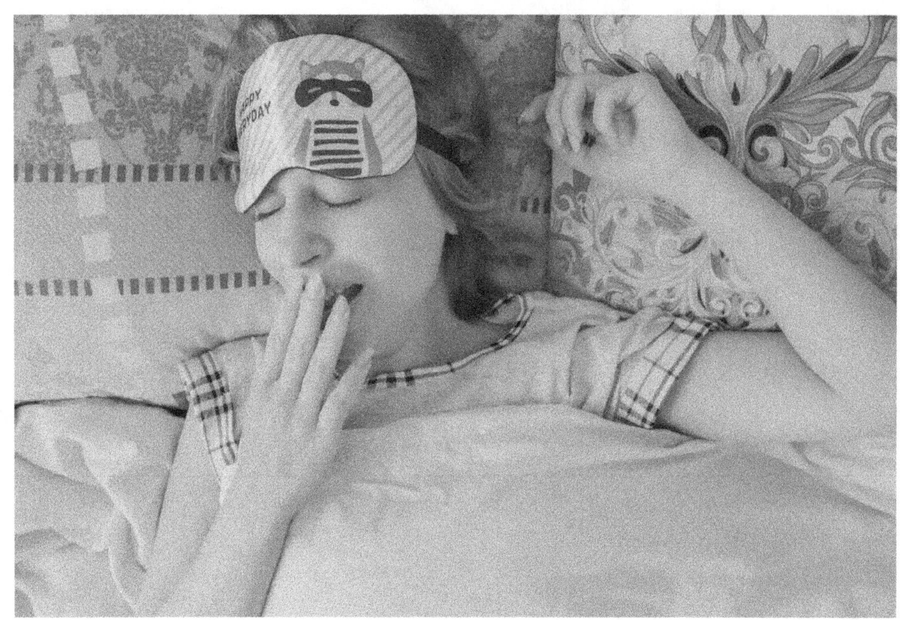

PLANNED COMMUNITIES. Due to accessibility or safety concerns, many people lack access to nearby locations to be active. A park is more than half a mile away from the majority of Americans' homes.

TRENDS IN CHILD CARE. Youngsters now play outside less frequently than they once did. Kids spend more time in childcare facilities that are enclosed and may not have enough room or equipment for physical activity. This is partially a result of societal tendencies that believe it is unsafe for kids to play outside unsupervised. Inadequate access to quality childcare and public areas are other contributing factors. In many daycare settings, free play is substituted for watching TV.

DISABILITY. Obesity is particularly common in adults and kids with physical and learning difficulties. Physical restrictions and a lack of sufficient resources and specialized education can both play a role.

CHAPTER 3: THE IMPORTANCE OF A HEALTHY DIET

One of the most important ways to drop fat now is by maintaining a healthy diet. A healthy diet can help you lose weight and reduce body fat. In this chapter, we will discuss the importance of a healthy diet and how to create a balanced meal plan that can help you achieve your weight loss goals.

All of the major food groups, including lean proteins, whole grains, healthy fats, and colorful fruits and vegetables, are typically represented in a healthy diet by nutrient-dense foods. Trans fats, added salt, and sugar-containing meals should be swapped out for more nutrient-dense alternatives as part of healthy eating practices.

A nutritious diet has several advantages, such as strengthening bones, defending the heart, preventing sickness, and elevating mood.

The top cause of death for people in the United States is heart disease, according to the Centers for Disease Control and Prevention (CDC)Trusted Source. About half of American adults, according to the American Heart Association (AHA)Trusted Source, have a cardiovascular illness.

In the US, high blood pressure, or hypertension, is becoming a bigger problem. An attack on the heart, cardiac failure, or a stroke can result from the condition.

Through lifestyle modifications, such as increasing physical exercise and eating healthily, it may be feasible to prevent up to 80% of early heart disease and stroke diagnoses.
People's diets can lower their blood pressure and support the health of their hearts.

People's diets can lower their blood pressure and support the health of their hearts.

The Dietary Approaches to Stop Hypertension (DASH) diet has a lot of heart-healthy foods.
- Consuming a lot of fruits, veggies, and whole grains

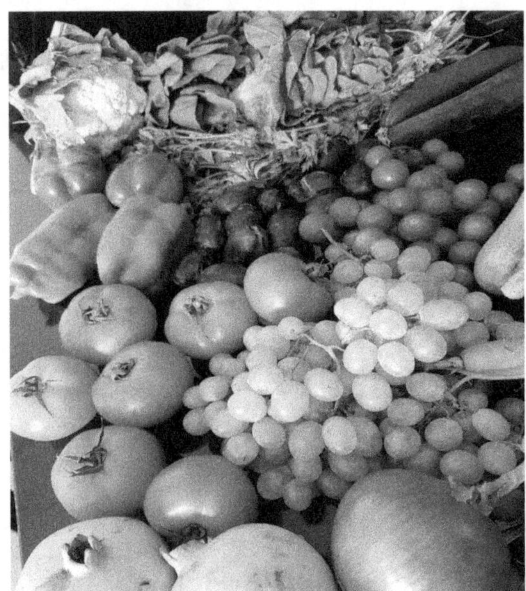

- selecting dairy products, fish, poultry, legumes, nuts, and vegetable oils that are low in fat or fat-free.

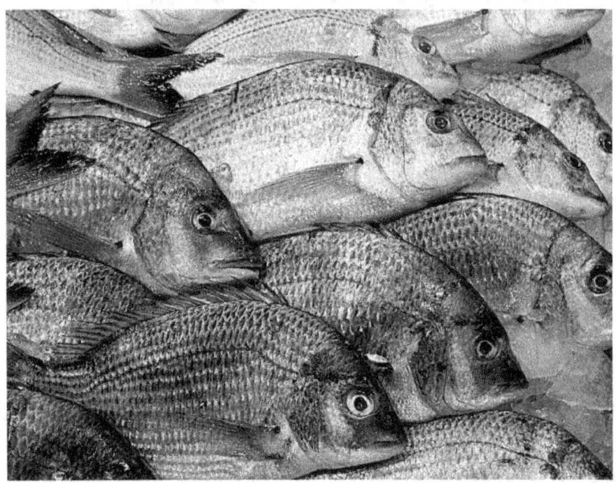

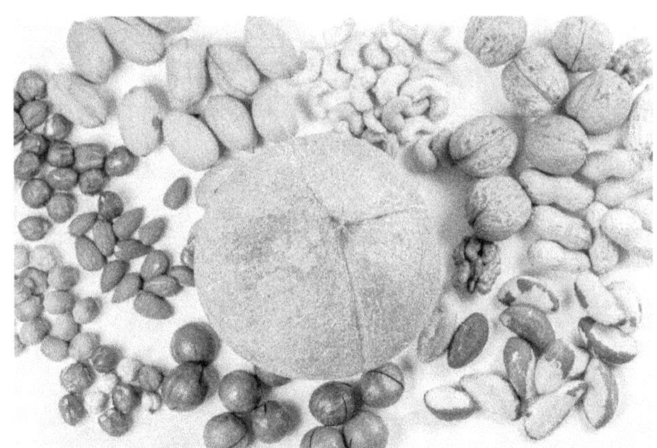

- Minimizing consumption of saturated and trans fats, such as those found in full-fat dairy and rich meats.

- Reducing intake of beverages and foods with added sugars.

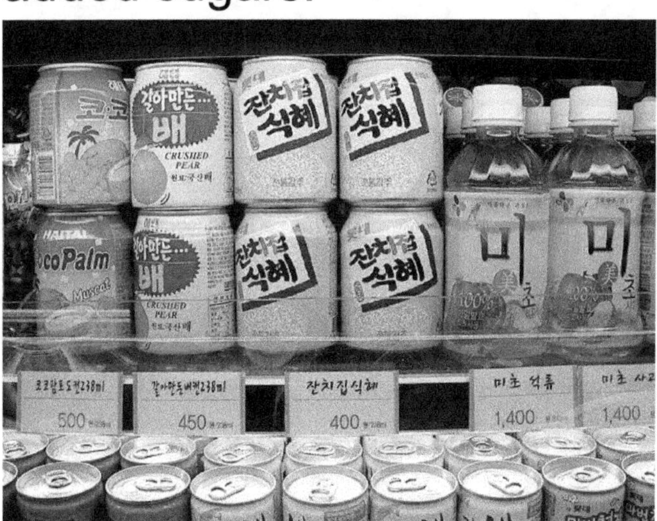

- Limiting daily salt intake to less than 2,300 milligrams, ideally 1,500 mg, and increasing potassium, magnesium, and calcium intake.

QUICK DIET RECOMMENDATIONS

There are many simple ways to enhance one's diet, such as:

- Substituting water or herbal tea for soda
- Making fresh produce a part of every meal and choosing healthy grains over processed ones
- Eating entire fruits as opposed to juice
- Reducing consumption of processed and red meats, which are heavy in salt and may raise the risk of colon cancer
- Adding additional lean protein to one's diet, which can be found in foods like eggs, tofu, salmon, and nuts
- Taking a cooking lesson and learning how to include more vegetables in meals can also be helpful.

CHAPTER 4: UNDERSTANDING CALORIES IN YOUR FOOD

Calories are the unit of energy in food. Understanding how many calories you need each day and how many you consume can help you lose weight and drop fat now.

The Unknown Factor in a Healthy Diet
There is a wealth of knowledge available regarding a healthy diet. It's circulated among friends and family, available in bookstores, and on the internet. You might believe that since there is so much knowledge available, becoming a health expert should be simple. Instead, the abundance of information can be overwhelming and confusing. This may be the case because calories, the most fundamental unit of food, are similarly cloaked in obscurity. Thus the first step to making wise, healthy decisions is to understand calories.

You can be too hungry when you sit down for a dinner to consider whether it is a balanced one. Or perhaps you adhere to the philosophy that "ignorance is bliss." Whatever the situation, knowledge is strength.

You may prepare meals that are well-balanced by learning the fundamentals of macronutrients and the number of calories they give. You can live the healthiest life possible by arming yourself with appropriate nutritional knowledge.

CHAPTER 5: THE ROLE OF EXERCISE IN WEIGHT LOSS VS DIET

Exercise is essential for weight loss and reducing body fat. A healthier diet and regular exercise are both better for weight loss than calorie restriction alone. Some diseases' consequences can be avoided or even reversed by exercise. Exercise reduces cholesterol and blood pressure, which may help to ward against a heart attack.

Also, exercising reduces your risk of getting some malignancies, like colon and breast cancer. Exercise is also known to support feelings of confidence and wellbeing, perhaps reducing anxiety and depressive symptoms.

Exercise aids in weight loss and weight maintenance. Exercise can boost metabolism, which is the amount of calories you burn each day. Lean body mass can be maintained and increased, which also contributes to a daily calorie burn increase.

HOW MUCH EXERCISE IS NEEDED TO LOSE WEIGHT?

It is advised that you engage in some type of aerobic exercise at least three times a week for a minimum of 20 minutes per session if you want to benefit from exercise's health benefits. If you want to genuinely reduce weight, it's best to exercise for longer than 20 minutes. A daily regimen of just 15 minutes of moderate activity, such as walking a mile, can result in a 100-calorie calorie burn (provided you don't eat too many calories afterward). During the course of a year, burning 700 calories each week can result in weight loss of up to 10 pounds.

HOW TO DETERMINE YOUR GOAL HEART RATE

You must mix in some higher intensity workouts if you want to reap the full range of health advantages from exercise. You may measure your heart rate to determine how hard you are working. The simplest method for calculating your desired heart rate is to remove your age from 220, then divide that result by 60 to 80 percent.

To find your ideal intensity for each workout, see a trainer or your medical team. Before starting any fitness program, anyone with unique health problems like an injury, diabetes, or a heart condition should speak with a doctor.

WHAT ARE A FEW EXAMPLES OF THE MANY WORKOUT FORMS?

What you select to exercise for weight loss is less important than whether or not you do it. For this reason, experts advise choosing exercises you enjoy in order to maintain a regular schedule.

AEROBIC

Whichever fitness regimen you choose to follow should contain some sort of aerobic or cardiovascular activity. Exercises that are aerobic increase heart rate and blood circulation. Exercises that are aerobic include cycling, swimming, dancing, walking, and jogging. You can exercise with a fitness machine like a stair stepper, elliptical, or treadmill.

WEIGHT TRAINING

Gaining muscle while exercising with weights has many benefits, including helping you lose fat. In turn, muscle burns calories. What a positive feedback cycle! All major muscle groups should be worked out three times per week, according to experts. This comprises:

abs
back
biceps
calves
 chest
forearms
hamstrings
quads
shoulders
traps
triceps

YOGA

According to a recent study by researchers at the Fred Hutchinson Cancer Research Center, yoga is not as rigorous as other forms of exercise, but it can still aid in weight loss in other ways. According to the study, those who practice yoga are less likely to be obese because they are more conscious of what they consume.

MAKING FITNESS A PART OF YOUR LIFESTYLE

More important than whether or not you exercise in a particular session is the total quantity of activity you get in a day. Because of this, even little adjustments to your everyday routine can have a significant impact on your waistline.

Following a healthy lifestyle includes the following:

While conducting errands, using the stairs rather than the elevator, parking further away from destinations, and then walking the entire distance

CONCLUSION

It can be challenging to create a healthy routine that includes exercise and balanced meals. Being aware of calories can be very beneficial. And fortunately, there are lots of tools at your disposal to make this process simpler. Find out first what your energy requirements are depending on your age, sex, weight, and degree of activity. This provides you with a strong foundation.

To make informed selections based on the labels on the food packaging, gather as much information as you can. By planning your meals and snacks in this way, you can meet your daily calorie needs. You may then determine how many calories you should be ingesting daily relative to your minimum energy requirements based on your weight management goals.

Decide how many calories you can burn based on the exercises you like to do. This can help you determine how frequently and for how long you should work out in order to reach your weight-management objectives.

The first step to becoming healthier may be to better understand calories. Whatever your objectives for health and fitness may be, you are more equipped to make choices now.